Sous Vide Cookbook for Beginners

Quick & Easy Recipes for Novice, Learn the Basic Techniques and start cook faster and smarter. Lose Weight and Boost metabolism with Effortless Everyday Meals

Frank Kimmons

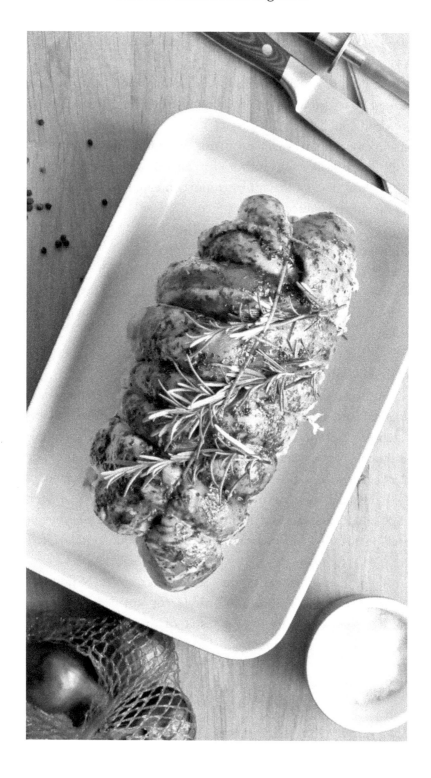

Table of Contents

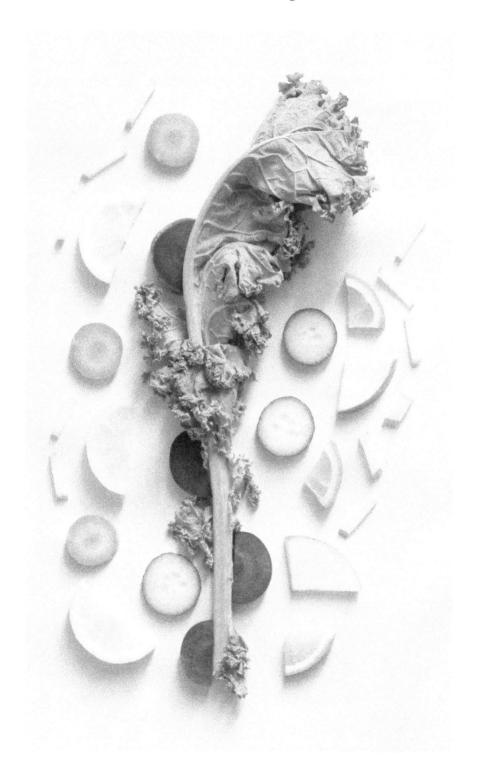

CHAPTER 1.   Red Meats

1. Cilantro-Garlic Beef Roast

Prep + Cook Time: 24 hours 30 minutes | Servings: 6

Ingredients

- 4 tbsp olive oil
- 2 pounds beef chuck
- Salt and black pepper to taste
- 1 tsp thyme
- 1 tsp cilantro
- 1 cup soy sauce
- ½ cup freshly squeezed lemon juice
- ½ cup freshly squeezed orange juice
- ½ cup Worcestershire sauce
- ¼ cup yellow mustard
- 3 garlic cloves, minced

Directions

Prepare a water bath and place the Sous Vide in it. Set to 141 F. Prepare the roast and truss it using butcher's twine. Season with salt, pepper, thyme, and cilantro. Put a pan over high heat. In the meantime, baste the roast with 2 tablespoons of olive oil using a soft brush. Place the meat on the pan to sear for 1 minute on both sides. Combine Worcestershire sauce, mustard, garlic, soy sauce, lemon and orange juice in one vessel.

Slide the beef in a vacuum-bag, mix it with the previously made marinade and close the bag using water displacement method. Cook in the water bath for 24 hours.

Once ready, open the bag and pour the liquid over to a small saucepan. Cook for 10 minutes over high heat until you reach half of the volume. Add 2 tablespoons of olive oil and preheat the iron-cast pan over high heat. Gently put the meat on the pan and sear one minute each side. Take the roast out of the pan and let cool down for about 5 minutes. Slice and add the sauce on top.

2. Beef Rib Eye Steak

Prep + Cook Time: 1 hour 40 minutes | Servings: 2

Ingredients

- 1 tbsp butter
- 1 pound rib-eye steak
- Salt and black pepper to taste
- ½ tsp garlic powder
- ½ tsp onion powder ½ tsp thyme

Directions

Prepare a water bath and place the Sous Vide in it. Set to 134 F. Rub both sides of the meat with salt, pepper, thyme, onion, and garlic powder. Slide into pieces inside the vacuum-bag, adding butter. Use water displacement method to seal the bag and put into the water bath. Cook for 90 minutes.

Once ready, get rid of the cooking liquid and take the steak out of the bag to pat dry with kitchen towel. Heat a cast-iron pan over high heat. Cook the steak for 1 minute per side. Let cool for 5 minutes before slicing.

3. Tasty Mediterranean Meatballs

Prep + Cook Time: 1 hour 55 minutes | Servings: 4

Ingredients

- 1 pound ground beef
- ½ cup bread crumbs
- ¼ cup milk
- 1 egg, beaten
- tbsp chopped fresh basil
- 1 garlic clove, minced
- 1 tsp salt
- ½ tsp dried basil
- 1 tbsp sesame oil

Directions

Prepare a water bath and place the Sous Vide in it. Set to 141 F. Combine beef, bread crumbs, milk, egg, basil, garlic, salt, and basil and shape into 14-16 meatballs. Place 6 meatballs in each vacuumsealable bag. Release air by the water displacement method, seal and submerge the bags in the water bath. Cook for 90 minutes. Heat the oil in a skillet over medium heat. Once the timer has stopped, remove the meatballs and transfer to the skillet and sear for 4-5 minutes.

Discard the cooking juices. Serve.

4. Traditional French-Style Steak

Prep + Cook Time: 2 hours 25 minutes | Servings: 5

Ingredients

- 4 tbsp butter
- 2 pounds sirloin steak
- Salt and black pepper to taste
- 2 shallot, chopped
- 1 fresh sage sprigs
- 1 fresh rosemary sprig

Directions

Prepare a water bath and place the Sous Vide in it. Set to 134 F. Melt 2 tablespoons of butter in a large cast-iron pan on high heat. Put the sirloin steak on the pan and sear each side for 30 to 45 seconds. Set the meat aside. Add the shallot, sage, and rosemary. Stir in butter and herbs. Cook for about 1-2 minutes until it gets bright green and soft. Slide the sirloin steak into a vacuum-bag, adding previously mixed herbs and seal the bag using the water displacement method. Cook for 2 hours.

Once ready, remove the meat and discard the cooking liquid. Put the sirloin steak on a plate lined with a paper towel or a baking sheet. Heat a cast-iron pan over high heat and add 2 tbsp of butter. When the butter sizzles, return the steak and sear for 2 minutes on both sides. Turn off the heat and leave the sirloin steak for about 5 minutes. Finally, cut into tiny pieces. Best served with vegetables and potatoes.

5. Yummy Smoked Beef Brisket

Prep + Cook Time: 33 hours 50 minutes | Servings: 8

Ingredients

- ¼ tsp liquid hickory smoke
- 8 tbsp honey
- Salt and black pepper to taste
- 1 tsp chili powder
- 1 tsp dried parsley
- 1 tsp garlic powder
- 1 tsp onion powder
- ½ tsp ground cumin
- 4 pounds beef brisket

Directions

Prepare a water bath and place the Sous Vide in it. Set to 156 F. Combine the honey, salt, pepper, chili powder, parsley, onion and garlic powder, and cumin. Reserve 1/4 of the mixture. Brush the brisket with the mixture. Place the brisket in a sizeable vacuumsealable bag with the liquid smoke. Release air by the water displacement method, seal, and submerge the bag in the water bath. Cook for 30 hours. Once the timer has stopped, remove the bag and allow to chill for 1 hour. Preheat the oven to 300 F. Pat dry with kitchen towels the brisket and brush with the reserved sauce. Discard the cooking juices.

Transfer the brisket to a baking tray, put into the oven and roast for 2 hours. Once the time has stopped, remove the brisket and cover it with aluminium foil for 40 minutes. Serve with baked beans, fresh bread, and butter.

6. Perfect Roast Steak

Prep + Cook Time: 20 hours 20 minutes | Servings: 4

Ingredients

- 4 tbsp sesame oil
- 4 chuck tender roast steaks
- 1 tsp garlic powder
- 1 tsp onion powder
- 1 tsp dried parsley
- Salt and black pepper to taste

Directions

Prepare a water bath and place the Sous Vide in it. Set to 130 F. Heat the sesame oil in a skillet over high heat and sear the steaks for 1 minute per side. Set aside and allow to cool. Combine the garlic powder, onion powder, parsley, salt and pepper. Rub the steaks with the mixture and place into a vacuum-sealable bag. Release air by the water displacement method, seal, and submerge the bag in the water bath. Cook for 20 hours. Once the timer has stopped, remove the steaks and pat dry with kitchen towel.

Discard the cooking juices.

7. Chipotle Beef Steak Coffee Rub

Prep + Cook Time: 1 hour 55 minutes | Servings: 4

Ingredients

- 1 tbsp olive oil
- 2 tbsp butter
- 1 tbsp sugar
- Salt and black pepper to taste
- 1 tbsp coffee grounds
- 1 tbsp garlic powder
- 1 tbsp onion powder
- 1 tbsp chipotle powder
- 4 strip steaks

Directions

Prepare a water bath and place the Sous Vide in it. Set to 130 F. Combine brown sugar, salt, pepper, coffee grounds, onion, garlic powder, and paprika in a small bowl. Place the steaks on the previously cleaned surface and brush a thin layer of olive oil. Place the steaks into separate vacuum-bags. Then close the bags using the water displacement method. Put into the water bath and cook them for 1 hour, 30 minutes.

Once ready, remove the steaks and discard the liquid. Put the steaks on a plate lined with a paper towel or a baking sheet. Heat a cast-iron pan over high heat and add butter. When the butter sizzles, put the tenderloin on the pan again and sear for 1 minute on both sides. Let cool for 2-3 minutes and slice to serve.

8. French-Style Stuffed Beef Burgers

Prep + Cook Time: 50 minutes | Servings: 5

Ingredients

- 1 egg
- 1 pound ground beef
- 3 green onions, chopped
- 2 tsp Worcestershire sauce
- 2 tsp soy sauce
- Salt and black pepper to taste
- 5 slices Camembert cheese
- 5 burger buns
- Iceberg lettuce leaves
- 5 tomato slices

Directions

Prepare a water bath and place the Sous Vide in it. Set to 134 F. Combine the beef, onion, egg, and soy sauce using your hands and season with salt and pepper. Shape the mixture into 8 patties. Place 1 cheddar slice in the center of each patty and place another patty over the cheddar. Combine well to create a single patty. Place the cheesy patties in four vacuum-sealable bags. Release air by the water displacement method, seal and submerge the bags in the water bath. Cook for 30 minutes. Once the timer has stopped, remove the patties and pat dry with a kitchen towel. Discard the cooking juices. Heat a skillet over high heat and sear the patties for 1 minute per side. Put the burgers over the toast buns. Top with lettuce and tomato.

9. Herby Skirt Steak

Prep + Cook Time: 3 hours 20 minutes | Servings: 6

Ingredients

- 2 tbsp butter
- 3 pounds skirt steak
- 2 tbsp extra-virgin oil
- 1 ½ tsp garlic powder
- Salt and black pepper to taste
- ¼ tsp onion powder
- ¼ tsp cayenne pepper
- ¼ tsp dried parsley
- ¼ tsp dried sage
- ¼ tsp crushed dried rosemary

Directions

Prepare a water bath and place the Sous Vide in it. Set to 134 F. Brush the steak with olive oil. Combine the garlic powder, salt, pepper, onion powder, cayenne pepper, parsley, sage, and rosemary. Rub the steak with the mixture.

Place the steak in a large vacuum-sealable bag. Release air by the water displacement method, seal, and submerge the bag in the water bath. Cook for 3 hours. Once the timer has stopped, remove the steak and pat dry with kitchen towel.

Heat the butter in a skillet over high heat and sear the steak for 2-3 minutes on all sides. Allow to rest for 5 minutes and cut to serve.

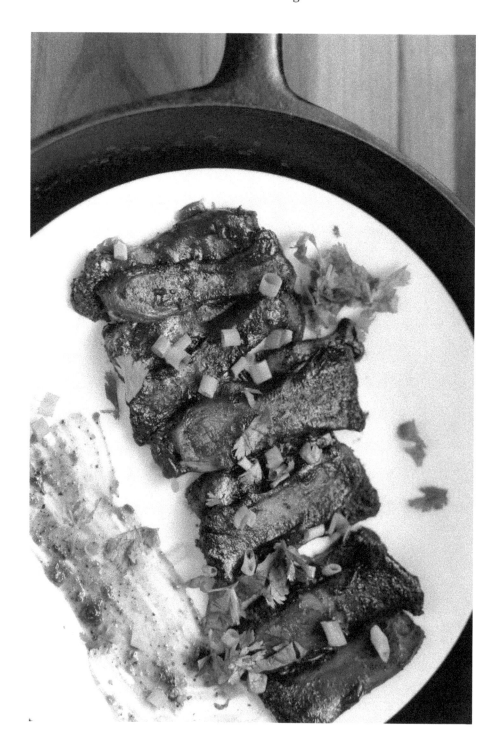

CHAPTER 2.   Pork

10.Sweet Mustard Pork with Crispy Onions

Prep + Cook Time: 48 hours 40 minutes | Servings: 6

Ingredients

- 1 tbsp ketchup
- 4 tbsp honey mustard
- 2 tbsp soy sauce
- 2 ¼ pounds pork shoulder
- 1 large sweet onion, cut into thin rings
- 2 cups milk
- 1 ½ cups all-purpose flour
- 2 tsp granulated onion powder
- 1 tsp paprika
- Salt and black pepper to taste
- 4 cups vegetable oil, for frying

Directions

Prepare a water bath and place the Sous Vide in it. Set to 159 F. Combine well the mustard, soy sauce and ketchup to make a paste. Brush the pork with the sauce and place in a vacuum-sealable bag.

Release air by the water displacement method, seal, and submerge the bag in the water bath. Cook for 48 hours. To make the onions: separate the onion rings in a bowl. Pour the milk over them and allow to chill for 1 hour. Combine the flour, onion powder, paprika, salt, and pepper. Heat the oil in a skillet over medium heat. Drain the onions and deepen in the flour mix. Shake well and transfer into the skillet. Fry them for 2 minutes or until gets crispy. Transfer to a baking sheet and pat dry with kitchen towel. Repeat the process with the remaining onions. Once the timer has stopped, remove the pork and transfer to a cutting board and pull the pork until it is shredded. Reserve cooking juices and transfer into a saucepan hot over medium heat and cook for 5 minutes until reduced. Top the pork with the sauce and garnish with crispy onions to serve.

11. Delicious Basil & Lemon Pork Chops

Prep + Cook Time: 1 hour 15 minutes | Servings: 4

Ingredients

- 4 tbsp butter
- 4 boneless pork rib chops
- Salt and black pepper to taste
- Zest and juice of 1 lemon
- 2 garlic cloves, smashed
- 2 bay leaves - 1 fresh basil sprig

Directions

Prepare a water bath and place the Sous Vide in it. Set to 141 F Season the chops with salt and pepper. Place the chops with the lemon zest and juice, garlic, bay leaves, basil, and 2 tbsp of butter in a vacuum-sealable bag. Release air by the water displacement method, seal, and submerge the bag in the water bath. Cook for 1 hour. Once the timer has stopped, remove the chops and pat dry with kitchen towel. Reserve the herbs. Heat the remaining butter in a skillet over medium heat and sear for 1-2 minutes per side.

12.Boneless Pork Ribs with Coconut-Peanut Sauce

Prep + Cook Time: 8 hours 30 minutes | Servings: 3

Ingredients

- ½ cup coconut milk
- 2 ½ tbsp peanut butter
- 2 tbsp soy sauce
- 1 tbsp sugar
- 3 inches fresh lemongrass
- 1 ½ tbsp pepper sauce
- 1 ½ inch ginger, peeled
- 3 cloves garlic
- 2 ½ tsp sesame oil
- 13 oz boneless pork ribs

Directions

Prepare a water bath and place Sous Vide in it. Set to 135 F. Blend all listed ingredients in a blender, except for the ribs and cilantro, until a smooth paste is obtained. Place the ribs and the mixture in a vacuumsealable bag. Release air by the water displacement method and seal the bag. Place in the water bath. Set the timer to 8 hours.

13. Baby Ribs with Chinese Sauce

Prep + Cook Time: 4 hours 25 minutes | Servings: 4

Ingredients

- 1/3 cup hoisin sauce
- 1/3 cup dark soy sauce
- 1/3 cup sugar
- 3 tbsp honey
- 3 tbsp white vinegar
- 1 tbsp fermented bean paste
- 2 tsp sesame oil
- 2 crushed garlic cloves
- 1-inch piece fresh grated ginger
- 1 ½ tsp five-spice powder
- Salt to taste
- ½ tsp fresh ground black pepper
- 3 pounds baby back ribs
- Cilantro leaves for serving

Directions

Prepare a water bath and place the Sous Vide in it. Set to 168 F. In a bowl, mix hoisin sauce, dark soy sauce, sugar, white vinegar, honey, bean paste, sesame oil, five-spice powder, salt, ginger, white and black pepper. Reserve 1/3 of the mixture and allow chilling. Brush the ribs with the mixture and share among 3 vacuum-sealable bag. Release air by the water displacement method, seal and submerge the bags in the water bath. Cook for 4 hours.

Preheat the oven to 400 F. Once the timer has stopped, remove the ribs and brush with the remaining mixture. Transfer to a baking tray and put in the oven. Bake for 3 minutes. Take out and allow resting for 5 minutes. Cut the rack and top with cilantro. Serve and enjoy!

14.Jerk Pork Ribs

Prep + Cook Time: 20 hours 10 minutes | Servings: 6

Ingredients

- 5 lb (2) baby back pork ribs, full racks
- ½ cup jerk seasoning mix

Directions

Make a water bath, place Sous Vide in it, and set to 145 F. Cut the racks into halves and season them with half of jerk seasoning. Place the racks in separate vacuum-sealable racks. Release air by the water displacement method, seal and submerge the bags in the water bath. Set the timer to 20 hours.

Cover the water bath with a bag to reduce evaporation and add water every 3 hours to avoid the water drying out. Once the timer has stopped, remove and unseal the bag. Transfer the ribs to a foiled baking sheet and preheat a broiler to high. Rub the ribs with the remaining jerk seasoning and place them in the broiler. Broil for 5 minutes. Slice into single ribs. Serve and enjoy!

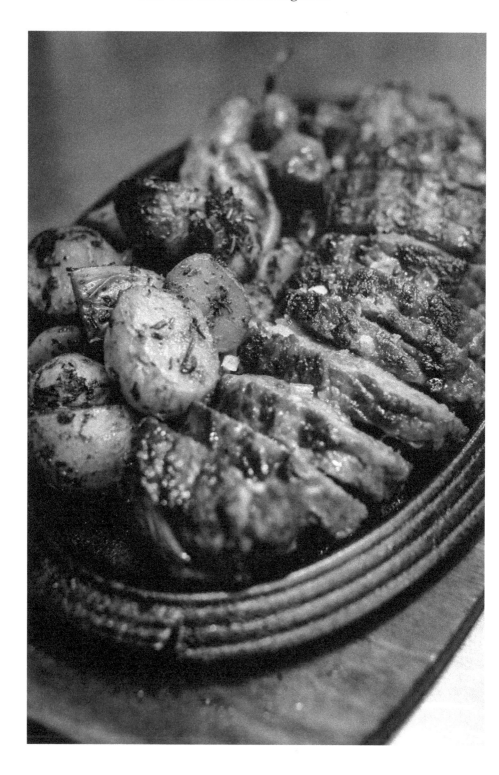

CHAPTER 3.   Poultry

15.Chili Chicken & Chorizo Tacos with Cheese

Prep + Cook Time: 3 hours 25 minutes | Servings: 6

Ingredients

- 2 pork sausages, casings removed
- 1 poblano pepper, stemmed and seeded
- ½ jalapeño pepper, stemmed
- 4 scallions, chopped
- 1 bunch fresh cilantro leaves
- ½ cup chopped fresh parsley
- 3 garlic cloves
- 2 tbsp lime juice
- 1 tsp salt
- ¾ tsp ground coriander
- ¾ tsp ground cumin
- 4 chicken breasts, sliced
- 1 tbsp vegetable oil
- ½ yellow onion, sliced thinly

- 8 corn taco shells

- 3 tbsp Provolone cheese

- 1 tomato

- 1 Iceberg lettuce, shredded

Directions

Put the ½ cup water, poblano pepper, jalapeño pepper, scallions, cilantro, parsley, garlic, lime juice, salt, coriander, and cumin in a blender and mix until smooth. Place the chicken strips and pepper mixture in a vacuum-sealable bag. Transfer to the fridge and allow to chill for 1 hour.

Prepare a water bath and place Sous Vide in it. Set to 141 F. Place the chicken mix in the bath. Cook for 1 hour and 30 minutes. Heat oil in a skillet over medium heat and sauté onion for 3 minutes. Add in chorizo and cook for 5-7 minutes. Once the timer has stopped, remove the chicken. Discard cooking juices. Add in chicken and mix well. Fill the tortillas with the chicken-chorizo mixture. Top with cheese, tomato and lettuce. Serve.

16. Easy Spicy-Honey Chicken

Prep + Cook Time: 1 hour 45 minutes | Servings: 4

Ingredients

- 8 tbsp butter
- 8 garlic cloves, chopped
- 6 tbsp chili sauce
- 1 tsp cumin
- 4 tbsp honey
- Juice of 1 lime
- Salt and black pepper to taste
- 4 boneless, skinless chicken breasts

Directions

Prepare a water bath and place the Sous Vide in it. Set to 141 F. Heat a saucepan over medium heat and put the butter, garlic, cumin, chili sauce, sugar, lime juice, and a pinch of salt and pepper. Cook for 5 minutes.

Combine the chicken with salt and pepper and place it in 4 vacuumsealable bag with the marinate. Release air by the water displacement method, seal and submerge the bags in the water bath. Cook for 1 hour and 30 minutes. Once the timer has stopped, remove the chicken and pat dry with kitchen towels. Reserve the half of cooking juices from each bag and transfer into a pot over medium heat. Cook until the sauce simmer, then Put the chicken inside and cook for 4 minutes. Remove the chicken and cut into slices. Serve with rice.

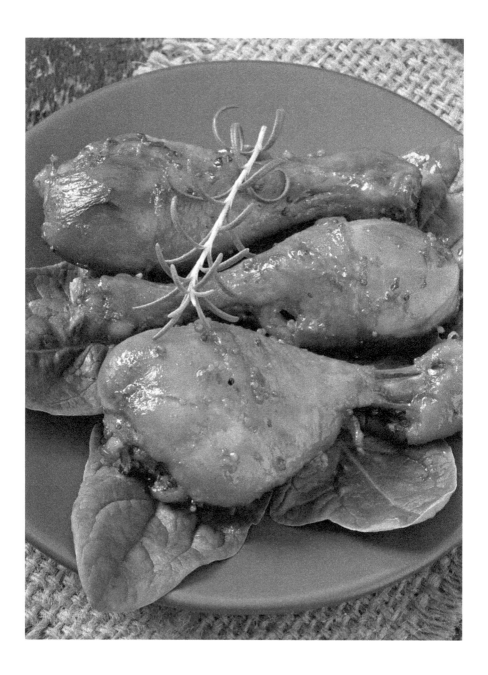

17.Crunchy Homemade Fried Chicken

Prep + Cook Time: 3 hours 20 minutes | Servings: 8

Ingredients

- ½ tbsp dried basil
- 2 ¼ cups sour cream
- 8 chicken drumsticks
- Salt and white pepper to taste
- ½ cup vegetable oil
- 3 cups flour
- 2 tbsp garlic powder
- 1 ½ tbsp Cayenne red pepper powder
- 1 tbsp dried mustard

Directions

Prepare a water bath and place the Sous Vide in it. Set to 156 F. Season the chicken salt and place in a vacuum-sealable bag. Release air by the water displacement method, seal and submerge in the water bath. Cook for 3 hours. Once the timer has stopped, remove the chicken and pat dry with kitchen towels.

Combine salt, flour, garlic powder, cayenne red pepper powders, mustard, white pepper, and basil in a bowl. Place sour cream in another bowl. Dip the chicken in the flour mixture, then in the sour cream and again in the flour mixture. Heat oil in a skillet over medium heat. Cook in the drumsticks for 3-4 minutes until crispy. Serve.

18. Classic Chicken Cordon Bleu

Prep + Cook Time: 1 hour 50 minutes + Cooling Time | Servings: 4

Ingredients

- ½ cup butter
- 4 boneless, skinless chicken breasts
- Salt and black pepper to taste
- 1 tsp cayenne pepper
- 4 garlic cloves, minced
- 8 ham slices
- 8 slices Emmental cheese

Directions

Prepare a water bath and place the Sous Vide in it. Set to 141 F. Season the chicken with salt and pepper. Cover with plastic wrap and rolled. Set aside and allow to chill.

Heat a saucepan over medium heat and add some black pepper, cayenne pepper, 1/4 cup of butter, and garlic. Cook until the butter melts. Transfer to a bowl. Rub the chicken on one side with the butter mixture. Then place 2 slices of ham and 2 slices of cheese and cover it. Roll each breast with plastic wrap and transfer to the fridge for 2-3 hours or in the freezer for 20-30 minutes.

Place the breast in two vacuum-sealable bags. Release air by the water displacement method, seal and submerge the bags in the water bath.

Cook for 1 hour and 30 minutes. Once done, remove the breasts and take off the plastic. Heat the remaining butter in a skillet over medium heat and sear the chicken for 1-2 minutes per side.

19.Spicy Chicken Breasts

Prep + Cook Time: 1 hour 40 minutes | Servings: 4

Ingredients

- ½ cup chili sauce - 2 tbsp butter
- 1 tbsp white vinegar
- 1 tbsp champagne vinegar
- 4 chicken breasts, halved
- Salt and black pepper to taste

Directions

Prepare a water bath and place the Sous Vide in it. Set to 141 F. Heat a saucepan over medium heat and combine the chili sauce, 1 tbsp of butter and vinegar. Cook until the butter melted. Set aside. Season the chicken with salt and pepper and place in two vacuumsealable bags with the chili mix. Release air by the water displacement method, seal and submerge the bags in the water bath. Cook for 1 hour and 30 minutes. Once the timer has stopped, remove the chicken and transfer to a baking sheet. Discard cooking juices. Heat the remaining butter in a skillet over high heat and sear the chicken 1 minute per side. Cut into stripes. Serve.

20.   Delicious Chicken Wings with Buffalo Sauce

Prep + Cook Time: 3 hours | Servings: 3

Ingredients

- 3 pounds capon chicken wings
- 2½ cups buffalo sauce
- 1 bunch fresh parsley

Directions

Prepare a water bath and place the Sous Vide in it. Set to 148 F. Combine the capon wings with salt and pepper. Place it in a vacuumsealable bag with 2 cups of buffalo sauce. Release air by the water displacement method, seal, and submerge the bag in the water bath. Cook for 2 hours. Heat the oven to broil. Once the timer has stopped, remove the wings and transfer them into a bowl. Pour the remaining buffalo sauce and mix well. Transfer the wings to a baking tray with aluminium foil and cover with the remaining sauce. Bake for 10 minutes, turning at least once. Garnish with parsley.

21. Savory Lettuce Wraps with Ginger-Chili Chicken

Prep + Cook Time: 1 hour 45 minutes | Servings: 5

Ingredients

- ½ cup hoisin sauce
- ½ cup sweet chili sauce
- 3 tbsp soy sauce
- 2 tbsp grated ginger
- 2 tbsp ground ginger
- 1 tbsp brown sugar
- 2 garlic cloves, minced
- Juice of 1 lime
- 4 chicken breasts, cubed
- Salt and black pepper to taste
- 12 lettuce leaves, rinsed
- ⅛ cup poppy seeds 4 chives

Directions

Prepare a water bath and place Sous Vide in it. Set to 141 F. Combine chili sauce, ginger, soy sauce, brown sugar, garlic, and half of the lime juice. Heat a saucepan over medium heat and pour in the mixture. Cook for 5 minutes. Set aside.

Season the breasts with salt and pepper. Place them in an even layer in a vacuum-sealable bag with the chili sauce mixture. Release air by the water displacement method, seal, and submerge the bag in the water bath. Cook for 1 hour and 30 minutes.

Once the timer has stopped, remove the chicken and pat dry with kitchen towels. Discard cooking juices. Combine the hoisin sauce with the chicken cubes and mix well. Make piles of 6 lettuce leaves.

Share chicken among lettuce leaves and top with the poppy seeds and chives before wrapping.

22.   Aromatic Lemon Chicken Breasts

Prep + Cook Time: 1 hour 50 minutes | Servings: 4

Ingredients

- 3 tbsp butter
- 4 boneless skinless chicken breasts
- Salt and black pepper to taste
- Zest and juice of 1 lemon
- ¼ cup heavy cream
- 2 tbsp chicken broth
- 1 tbsp chopped fresh sage leaves
- 1 tbsp olive oil
- 3 garlic cloves, minced
- 1/4 cup red onions, chopped
- 1 large lemon, thinly sliced

Directions

Prepare a water bath and place the Sous Vide in it. Set to 141 F. Season the breast with salt and pepper.

Heat a saucepan over medium heat and combine the lemon juice and zest, heavy cream, 2 tbsp of butter, chicken broth, sage, olive oil, garlic, and red onions. Cook until the butter has melted. Place the breasts in 2 vacuum-sealable bags with the lemon-butter mix. Add in lemon slices. Release air by the water displacement method, seal and submerge the bags in the bath. Cook for 90 minutes.

Once the timer has stopped, remove the breasts and pat dry with kitchen towels. Discard the cooking juices. Heat the remaining butter in a skillet and sear the breasts for 1 minute per side. Cut the breasts into strips. Serve.

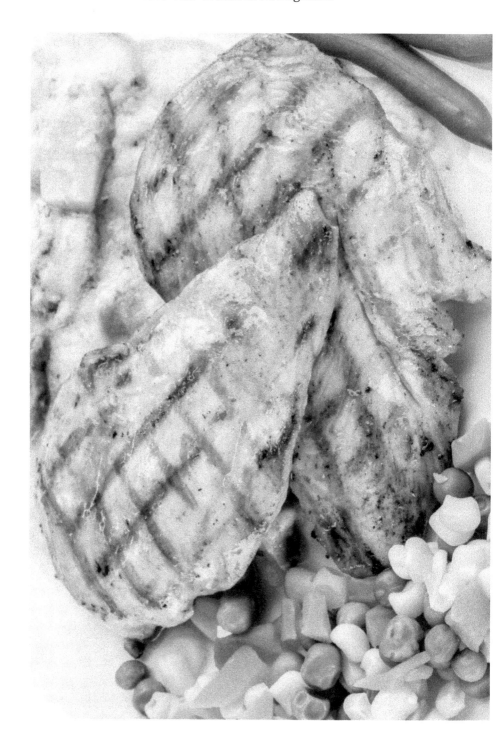

CHAPTER 4.   Fish & Seafood

23.   Halibut with Sweet Sherry & Miso Glaze

Prep + Cook Time: 50 minutes | Servings: 4

Ingredients

- 1 tbsp olive oil
- 2 tbsp butter
- ⅓ cup sweet sherry
- ⅓ cup red miso
- ¼ cup mirin
- 3tbsp brown sugar
- 2½ tbsp soy sauce
- 4 fillets halibut
- 2 tbsp chopped scallions
- 2 tbsp chopped fresh parsley

Directions

Prepare a water bath and place the Sous Vide in it. Set to 134 F. Heat the butter in a saucepan over medium-low heat. Stir in sweet sherry, miso, mirin, brown sugar, and soy sauce for 1 minute. Set aside. Allow to cool. Place the halibut in 2 vacuum-sealable bags. Release air by the water displacement method, seal and submerge the bags in the water bath. Cook for 30 minutes.

Once the timer has stopped, remove the halibut from the bags and pat dry with kitchen towels. Reserve cooking juices. Heat a saucepan over high heat and pour in cooking juices. Cook until reduced by half.

Heat olive oil in a skillet over medium heat and transfer the fillets. Sear for 30 seconds on each side until crispy. Serve the fish and drizzle with Miso Glaze. Garnish with scallions and parsley.

24.   Crispy Salmon with Sweet Ginger Glaze

Prep + Cook Time: 53 minutes | Servings: 4

Ingredients

- ½ cup Worcestershire sauce
- 6 tbsp white sugar
- 4 tbsp mirin
- 2 small garlic cloves, minced
- ½ tsp cornstarch
- ½ tsp grated fresh ginger
- 4 salmon fillets
- 4 tsp vegetable oil
- 2 cups cooked rice, for serving
- 1 tsp toasted poppy seeds

Directions

Prepare a water bath and place the Sous Vide in it. Set to 129 F. Combine the Worcestershire sauce, sugar, mirin, garlic, cornstarch, and ginger in a pot over medium heat. Cook for 1 minute until the sugar has dissolved. Reserve 1/4 cup of sauce. Allow to cool. Place the fillets salmon in 2 vacuum-sealable bags with the remaining sauce.

Release air by the water displacement method, seal and submerge the bags in the bath. Cook for 40 minutes.

Once the timer has stopped, remove the fillets from the bags and pat dry with kitchen towels. Heat a saucepan over medium heat and cook the cup of sauce for 2 minutes until thickened. Heat oil in a skillet. Sear the salmon for 30 seconds per side. Serve salmon with sauce and poppy seeds.

25.   Tasty Trout with Tamari Sauce

Prep + Cook Time: 35 minutes | Servings: 4

Ingredients

- ¼ cup olive oil

- 4 trout fillets, skinned and sliced

- ½ cup Tamari sauce

- ¼ cup light brown sugar

- 2 garlic cloves, minced

- 1 tbsp Coleman's mustard

Directions

Prepare a water bath and place Sous Vide in it. Set to 130 F. Combine the Tamari sauce, brown sugar, olive oil, and garlic. Place the trout in a vacuum-sealable bag with tamari mixture. Release air by the water displacement method, seal, and submerge the bag in the bath. Cook for 30 minutes. Once the timer has stopped, remove the trout and pat dry with kitchen towels. Discard the cooking juices. Garnish with tamari sauce and mustard to serve.

26.　　Citrus Fish with Coconut Sauce

Prep time: 1 hour 57 minutes | Servings: 6

Ingredients

- 2 tbsp vegetable oil
- 4 tomatoes, peeled and chopped
- 2 red bell peppers, diced
- 1 yellow onion, diced
- ½ cup orange juice
- ¼ cup lime juice
- 4 garlic cloves, minced
- 1 tsp caraway seeds, crushed
- 1 tsp cumin powder
- 1 tsp cayenne pepper
- ½ tsp salt
- 6 cod fillets, skin removed, cubed
- 14 ounces coconut milk
- ¼ cup shredded coconut
- 3 tbsp chopped fresh cilantro

Directions

Prepare a water bath and place the Sous Vide in it. Set to 137 F.

Combine in a bowl, the orange juice, lime juice, garlic, caraway seeds, cumin, cayenne pepper, and salt. Brush the fillets with the lime mixture. Cover and allow to chill in the fridge for 1 hour.

Meantime, heat oil in a saucepan over medium heat and put in tomatoes, bell peppers, onion, and salt. Cook for 4-5 minutes until softened. Pour the coconut milk over the tomato mixture and cook for 10 minutes. Let cool.

Take out the fillets from the fridge and place them in 2 vacuumsealable bags with the coconut mixture. Release air by the water displacement method, seal and submerge the bags in the water bath. Cook for 40 minutes. Once the timer has stopped, remove the bags and transfer the contents into a serving bowl. Garnish with shredded coconut and cilantro. Serve with rice.

27.　　Lime-Parsley Poached Haddock

Prep + Cook Time: 75 minutes | Servings: 4

Ingredients

- 4 haddock fillets, skin on
- ½ tsp salt
- 6 tbsp butter
- Zest and juice of 1 lime
- 2 tsp chopped fresh parsley
- 1 lime, quartered

Directions

Prepare a water bath and place the Sous Vide in it. Set to 137 F.

Season the fillets with salt and place in 2 vacuum-sealable bags. Add butter, half the lime zest and lime juice, and 1 tbsp of parsley. Release air by the water displacement method. Transfer into the fridge and allow to chill for 30 minutes. Seal and submerge the bags in the water bath. Cook for 30 minutes.

Once the timer has stopped, remove the fillets and pat dry with kitchen towels. Heat the remaining butter in a skillet over medium heat and sear the fillets for 45 seconds on each side, spooning the melted butter over the top. Pat dry with kitchen towel and transfer to a plate.

Garnish with lime quarters and serve.

28. Crispy Tilapia with Mustard-Maple Sauce

Prep + Cook Time: 65 minutes | Servings: 4

Ingredients

- 2 tbsp maple syrup - 6 tbsp butter
- 2 tbsp Dijon mustard
- 2 tbsp brown sugar
- tablespoon parsley
- 1 tablespoon thyme
- 2 tbsp soy sauce
- tbsp white wine vinegar 4 tilapia fillets, skin on

Directions

Prepare a water bath and place the Sous Vide in it. Set to 114 F. Melt 4 tbsp butter in a pan over medium heat and stir-fry in mustard, brown sugar, maple syrup, soy sauce, vinegar, parsley, and thyme for 2 minutes. Let cool.

Place tilapia fillets in a vacuum-sealable bag with maple sauce. Release air by the water displacement method, seal, and submerge the bag in the water bath. Cook for 45 minutes. Once ready, remove the fillets and place them in a preheated with the remaining butter skillet. Sear them for 2 minutes. Serve topped with mustard sauce.

29.   Swordfish & Potato Salad with Kalamata Olives

Prep + Cook Time: 3 hours 5 minutes | Servings: 2

Ingredients

- Potatoes
- 3 tbsp olive oil
- 1 pound sweet potatoes
- 2 tsp salt
- 3 fresh thyme sprigs
- Fish
- 1 tbsp olive oil
- 1 swordfish steak
- Salt and black pepper to taste
- 1 tsp canola oil
- Salad
- 1 cup baby spinach leaves
- 1 cup cherry tomatoes, halved
- ¼ cup Kalamata olives, chopped
- 1 tbsp olive oil
- 1 tsp Dijon mustard
- 3 tbsp cider vinegar
- ¼ tsp salt

Directions

To make the potatoes: prepare a water bath and place the Sous Vide in it. Set to 192 F.

Place the potatoes, olive oil, sea salt and thyme in a vacuum-sealable bag. Release air by the water displacement method, seal, and submerge the bag in the water bath. Cook for 1 hour and 15 minutes. Once the timer has stopped, remove the bag and do not open. Set aside.

To make the fish: Make a water bath and place the Sous Vide in it. Set to 104 F. Season the swordfish with salt and pepper. Place in a vacuum-sealable bag with olive oil. Release air by the water displacement method, seal, and submerge the bag in the water bath. Cook for 30 minutes.

Heat canola oil in a skillet over high heat. Remove the swordfish and pat pat dry with kitchen towels. Discard the cooking juices. Transfer the swordfish into the skillet and cook for 30 seconds per side. Cut into slices and cover with plastic wrap. Set aside.

Finally, make the salad: to a salad bowl, add the cherry tomatoes, olives, olive oil, mustard, cider vinegar, and salt and mix well. Add in baby spinach. Remove the potatoes and cut themby the half. Discard cooking juices. Top the salad with potatoes and swordfish to serve.

30. Buttery Red Snapper with Citrus Saffron Sauce

Prep + Cook Time: 55 minutes | Servings: 4

Ingredients

- 4 pieces cleaned red snapper
- 2 tbsp butter
- Salt and black pepper to taste
- For Citrus Sauce
- 1 lemon
- 1 grapefruit
- 1 lime
- 3 oranges
- 1 tsp Dijon mustard
- 2 tbsp canola oil
- 1 yellow onion
- 1 diced zucchini
- 1 tsp saffron threads
- 1 tsp diced chili pepper
- 1 tbsp sugar
- 3 cups fish stock
- 3 tbsp chopped cilantro

Directions

Prepare a water bath and place the Sous Vide in it. Set to 132 F. Season the snapper fillets with salt and pepper and place in a vacuum-sealable bag. Release air by the water displacement method, seal, and submerge the bag in the water bath. Cook for 30 minutes.

Peel the fruits and chop in cubes. Heat oil in a skillet over medium heat and put the onion and zucchini. Sauté for 2-3 minutes. Add the fruits, saffron, pepper, mustard and sugar. Cook for 1 minute more. Stir the fish stock and simmer for 10 minutes. Garnish with cilantro, and set aside. Once the timer has stopped, remove the fish and transfer to a plate. Glaze with citrus-saffron sauce and serve.

CHAPTER 5.   Eggs

31.Ground Beef Omelet

Prep + Cook Time: 35 minutes | Servings: 3

Ingredients

- 1 cup lean ground beef
- ¼ cup finely chopped onions
- ¼ tsp dried thyme, ground
- ½ tsp dried oregano, ground
- Salt and black pepper to taste 1 tbsp olive oil

Directions :

Preheat the oil in a skillet over medium heat. Add onions and stir-fry for about 3-4 minutes, or until translucent. Add ground beef and cook for 5 minutes, stirring occasionally. Sprinkle with some salt, pepper, thyme, and oregano. Stir well and cook for a minute more. Remove from the heat and set aside.

Prepare a water bath and place the Sous Vide in it. Set to 170 F. Whisk the eggs in a medium bowl and pour in a vacuum-resealable bag. Add beef mixture.

Release air by the water displacement method and seal the bag.

Immerse the bag in the water bath and set the timer for 15 minutes. Using a glove, massage the bag every 5 minutes to ensure even cooking. Once the timer stopped, remove the bag from the water bath and transfer the omelet to a serving plate.

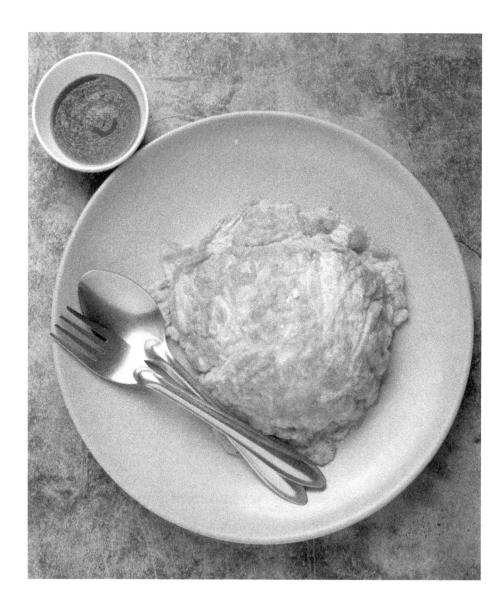

32.   Eggs in Bacon

Prep + Cook Time: 7 hours 15 minutes | Servings: 4

Ingredients

- 4 boiled eggs
- 1 tsp butter
- 7 ounces bacon, sliced
- 1 tbsp Dijon mustard
- 4 ounces mozzarella cheese, sliced
- Salt and black pepper to taste

Directions

Prepare a water bath and place the Sous Vide in it. Set to 140 F. Rub bacon with butter and pepper. Place a slice of mozzarella cheese on top of each egg and wrap the eggs along with the cheese in bacon. Brush with mustard and place them in a vacuum-sealable bag. Release air by the water displacement method, seal, and submerge the bag in the water bath. Set the timer for 7 hours. Once the timer has stopped, remove the bag and transfer to a plate. Serve warm.

CHAPTER 6.   Appetizers and Snacks

33.   Italian Chicken Fingers

Prep + Cook Time: 2 hours 20 minutes | Servings: 3

Ingredients

- 1 pound chicken breasts
- 1 cup almond flour
- tsp minced garlic - 1 tsp salt
- ½ tsp cayenne pepper
- 2 tsps mixed Italian herbs
- ¼ tsp black pepper
- eggs, beaten ¼ cup olive oil

Directions

Rinse the meat under cold running water and pat dry with kitchen paper. Season with mixed Italian herbs and place in a large vacuumsealable. Seal the bag and cook the chicken in sous vide for 2 hours at 167 F. Remove from the water bath and set aside. Now combine together flour, salt, cayenne, Italian herbs, and pepper in a bowl and set aside. In a separate bowl, beat the eggs and set aside. Heat olive oil in a large skillet, over medium heat. Dip the chicken into the beaten egg and coat with the flour mixture. Fry for 5 minutes on each side, or until golden brown.

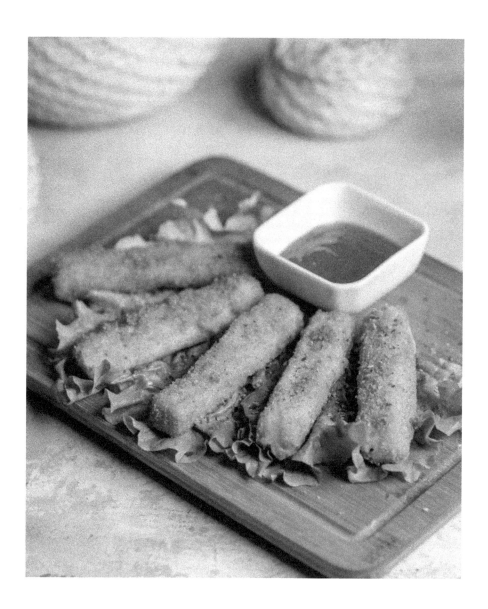

34.   Cherry Chicken Bites

Prep + Cook Time: 1 hour and 40 minutes | Servings: 3

Ingredients

- 1 pound chicken breast, boneless and skinless, cut into bite-sized pieces
- 1 red bell pepper, chopped into chunks
- 1 green bell pepper, chopped into chunks
- 1 cup cherry tomatoes, whole
- 1 cup olive oil
- 1 tsp Italian seasoning mix
- 1 tsp cayenne pepper
- ½ tsp dried oregano
- Salt and black pepper to taste

Directions

Rinse the meat under cold running water and pat dry with kitchen paper. Cut into bite-sized pieces and set aside. Wash the bell peppers and cut them into chunks. Wash the cherry tomatoes and remove the green stems. Set aside. In a bowl, combine olive oil with Italian seasoning, cayenne, salt, and pepper.

Stir until well incorporated. Add the meat and coat well with the marinade. Set aside for 30 minutes to allow flavors to meld and penetrate into the meat. Place the meat along with vegetables in a large vacuum-sealable bag. Add three tablespoons of the marinade and seal the bag. Cook in sous vide for 1 hour at 149 F.

35.   Herby Italian Sausage Pannini

Prep + Cook Time: 3 hours 15 minutes | Servings: 4

Ingredients

- 1 pound Italian sausage 1 red bell pepper, sliced
- 1 yellow bell pepper, sliced
- 1 onion, sliced
- 1 garlic clove, minced
- 1 cup tomato juice
- 1 tsp dried oregano
- 1 tsp dried basil
- 1 tsp olive oil
- Salt and black pepper to taste
- 4 bread slices

Directions

Prepare a water bath and place the Sous Vide in it. Set to 138 F. Place the sausages in a vacuum-sealable bag. Add the garlic, basil, onion, pepper, tomato juice, and oregano in each bag. Release air by the water displacement method, seal and submerge the bags in the water bath. Cook for 3 hours.

Once the timer has stopped, remove the sausages and transfer to a hot skillet. Fry them for 1 minute per side. Set aside. Add the remaining ingredients in the skillet, season with salt and pepper. Cook until water has evaporated. Serve the sausages and the remaining ingredients in between the bread.

36.   Cinnamon Persimmon Toast

Prep + Cook Time: 4 hours 10 minutes | Servings: 6

Ingredients

- 4 Bread Slices, toasted
- 4 Persimmons, chopped
- 3 tbsp Sugar
- ½ tsp Cinnamon
- 2 tbsp Orange Juice
- ½ tsp Vanilla Extract

Directions

Prepare a water bath and place the Sous Vide in it. Set to 155 F.

Place persimmons in a vacuum-sealable bag. Add in orange juice, vanilla extract, sugar, and cinnamon. Close the bag and shake well to coat the persimmon pieces. Release air by the water displacement method, seal, and submerge the bag in the water bath. Set the timer for 4 hours. Once the timer has stopped, remove the bag and transfer the persimmons to a food processor. Blend until smooth. Spread the persimmon mixture over bread.

37.   Chicken Wings with Ginger

Prep + Cook Time: 2 hours 25 minutes | Servings: 4

Ingredients

- 2 pounds chicken wings
- ¼ cup extra virgin olive oil
- 4 garlic cloves
- 1 tbsp rosemary leaves, finely chopped
- 1 tsp white pepper
- 1 tsp cayenne pepper
- 1 tbsp fresh thyme, finely chopped
- 1 tbsp fresh ginger, grated
- ¼ cup lime juice
- ½ cup apple cider vinegar

Directions

In a large bowl, combine olive oil with garlic, rosemary, white pepper, cayenne pepper, thyme, ginger, lime juice, and apple cider vinegar. Submerge wings in this mixture and cover. Refrigerate for one hour. Transfer the wings along with the marinade in a large vacuumsealable bag. Seal the bag and cook in sous vide for 1 hour and 15 minutes at 149 F. Remove from the vacuum-sealable bag and brown before serving. Serve and enjoy!

38.   Beef Patties

Prep + Cook Time: 1 hour 55 minutes | Servings: 4

Ingredients

- pound lean ground beef
- 1 egg
- 2 tbsp almonds, finely chopped
- tbsp almond flour
- 1 cup onions, finely chopped
- 2 garlic cloves, crushed
- ¼ cup olive oil
- Salt and black pepper to taste
- ¼ cup parsley leaves, finely chopped

Directions

In a bowl, combine ground beef with finely chopped onions, garlic, oil, salt, pepper, parsley, and almonds. Mix well with a fork and gradually add some almond flour. Whisk in one egg and refrigerate for 40 minutes. Remove the meat from the refrigerator and gently form into one-inch-thick patties, about 4-inches in diameter. Place in a two separate vacuum-sealable bags and cook in sous vide for one hour at 129 F.

CHAPTER 7.   Sauces, Stocks and Broths

39.   Spicy BBQ Sauce

Prep + Cook Time: 1 hour 15 minutes | Servings: 10

Ingredients

- 1 ½ lb small tomatoes
- ¼ cup apple cider vinegar
- ¼ tsp sugar
- 1 tbsp Worcestershire sauce
- ½ tbsp liquid hickory smoke
- 2 tsp smoked paprika
- 2 tsp garlic powder
- 1 tsp onion powder
- Salt to taste
- ½ tsp chili powder
- ½ tsp cayenne pepper
- 4 tbsp water

Directions

Make a water bath, place Sous Vide in it, and set to 185 F. Place the tomatoes into two vacuum-sealable bags. Release air by the water displacement method, seal and submerge the bags in the bath. Set the timer to 40 minutes.

Once the timer has stopped, remove and unseal the bags. Transfer the tomatoes to a blender and puree until smooth and thick.

Do not add water. Put a pot over medium heat, add in tomato puree and the remaining ingredients. Bring to a boil, stirring continuously for 20 minutes. A thick consistency should be achieved.

40.   Tomato Sauce

Prep + Cook Time: 55 minutes | Servings: 4

Ingredients

- 1 (16-oz) can tomatoes, crushed
- 1 small white onion, diced
- 1 cup fresh basil leaves
- 1 tbsp olive oil
- 1 clove garlic, crushed
- Salt to taste
- 1 bay leaf 1 red chili

Directions

Make a water bath, place Sous Vide in it, and set to 185 F. Place all the listed ingredients in a vacuum-sealable bag. Release air by the water displacement method, seal, and submerge the bag in the water bath. Set the timer for 40 minutes. Once the timer has stopped, remove and unseal the bag. Discard the bay leaf and transfer the remaining ingredients to a blender and puree smooth. Serve as a side sauce.

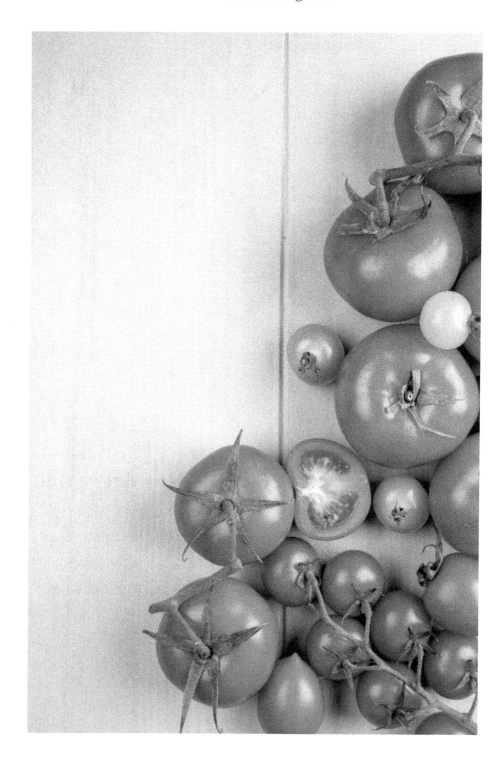

CHAPTER 8.   Vegetarian & Vegan

41.Cream of Tomatoes with Cheese Sandwich

Prep + Cook Time: 55 minutes | Servings: 8

Ingredients

- ½ cup cream cheese
- 2 pounds tomatoes, cut into wedges
- Salt and black pepper to taste
- 2 tbsp olive oil
- 2 garlic cloves, minced
- ½ tsp chopped fresh sage
- ⅛ tsp red pepper flakes
- ½ tsp white wine vinegar
- 2 tbsp butter
- 4 slices bread
- 2 slices halloumi cheese

Directions

Prepare a water bath and place the Sous Vide in it. Set to 186 F. Put the tomatoes in a colander over a bowl and season with salt. Stir well. Allow to chill for 30 minutes. Discard the juices. Combine the olive oil, garlic, sage, black pepper, salt, and pepper flakes. Place in a vacuum-sealable bag. Release air by the water displacement method, seal, and submerge the bag in the water bath. Cook for 40 minutes. Once the timer has stopped, remove the bag and transfer into a blender. Add in vinegar and cream cheese. Mix until smooth. Transfer to a plate and season with salt and pepper if needed.

To make the cheese bars: heat a skillet over medium heat. Grease the bread slices with butter and put into the skillet. Lay cheese slices over the bread and place over another buttery bread. Toast for 1-2 minutes. Repeat with the remaining bread. Cut into cubes. Serve over the warm soup.

42.   Garlic Tabasco Edamame Cheese

Prep + Cook Time: 1 hour 6 minutes | Servings: 4

Ingredients

- 1 tbsp olive oil
- 4 cups fresh edamame in pods
- 1 tsp salt
- 1 garlic clove, minced
- 1 tbsp red pepper flakes
- 1 tbsp Tabasco sauce

Directions

Prepare a water bath and place the Sous Vide in it. Set to 186 F. Heat a pot with water over high heat and blanch the edamame pots for 60 seconds. Strain them and transfer into an ice water bath. Combine the garlic, red pepper flakes, Tabasco sauce, and olive oil. Place the edamame in a vacuum-sealable bag. Pour the Tabasco sauce. Release air by the water displacement method, seal, and submerge the bag in the water bath. Cook for 1 hour. Serve and enjoy!

43.   Citrus Corn with Tomato Sauce

Prep + Cook Time: 55 minutes | Servings: 8

Ingredients

- ⅓ cup olive oil
- 4 ears yellow corn, husked
- Salt and black pepper to taste
- 1 large tomato, chopped
- 3 tbsp lemon juice
- 2 garlic cloves, minced
- 1 serrano pepper, seeded
- 4 scallions, green parts only, chopped
- ½ bunch fresh cilantro leaves, chopped

Directions

Prepare a water bath and place the Sous Vide in it. Set to 186 F. Whisk the corns with olive oil and season with salt and pepper. Place them in a vacuum-sealable bag. Release air by the water displacement method, seal, and submerge the bag in the water bath. Cook for 45 minutes.

Meantime, combine well the tomato, lemon juice, garlic, serrano pepper, scallions, cilantro, and the remaining olive oil in a bowl. Preheat a grill over high heat. Once the timer has stopped, remove the corns and transfer to the grill and cook for 2-3 minutes. Allow to cool. Cut the kernels from the cob and pour in tomato sauce. Serve.

44.   Sage Roasted Potato Mash

Prep + Cook Time: 1 hour 35 minutes | Servings: 6

Ingredients

- ¼ cup butter
- 12 sweet potatoes, unpeeled
- 10 garlic cloves, chopped
- 4 tsp salt
- 6 tbsp olive oil
- 5 fresh sage sprigs 1 tbsp paprika

Directions

Prepare a water bath and place the Sous Vide in it. Set to 192 F. Combine the potatoes, garlic, salt, olive oil and 2 or 3 thyme springs and place in a vacuum-sealable bag. Release air by the water displacement method, seal, and submerge the bag in the water bath. Cook for 1 hour and 15 minutes. Preheat the oven to 450 F. Once the timer has stopped, remove the potatoes and transfer into a bowl. Separate the cooking juices. Combine well the potatoes with butter and the remaining sage springs. Transfer into a baking tray, previously lined with aluminium foil. Make a hole in the center of the potatoes and pour the cooking juices in. Bake the potatoes for 10 minutes, turning 5 minutes later. Discard the sage. Serve sprinkled with paprika.

45.   Maple Beet Salad with Cashews & Queso Fresco

Prep + Cook Time: 1 hour 35 minutes | Servings: 8

Ingredients

- 6 large beets, cut into chunks
- Salt and black pepper to taste
- 3 tbsp maple syrup
- 2 tbsp butter
- Zest of 1 large orange
- 1 tbsp olive oil
- ½ tsp cayenne pepper
- 1 ½ cups cashews
- 6 cup arugula
- 3 tangerines, peeled and segmented
- 1 cup queso fresco, crumbled

Directions

Prepare a water bath and place the Sous Vide in it. Set to 186 F. Place the beet chunks in a vacuum-sealable bag. Season with salt and pepper. Add 2 tbsp of maple syrup, butter, and orange zest. Release air by the water displacement method, seal, and submerge the bag in the water bath. Cook for 1 hour and 15 minutes. Preheat the oven to 350 F. Mix the remaining maple syrup, olive oil, salt, and cayenne. Add in cashews and stir well. Transfer the cashew mixture into a baking tray, previously lined with wax pepper and bake for 10 minutes.

Allow to cool. Once the timer has stopped, remove the beets and discard the cooking juices. Put the arugula on a serving plate, beets, and tangerine wedges all over. Scatter with queso fresco and cashew mix to serve.

46.　　　Celery & Leek Potato Soup

Prep + Cook Time: 2 hours 15 minutes | Servings: 8

Ingredients

- 8 tbsp butter
- 4 red potatoes, sliced
- 1 yellow onion, cut into ¼-inch pieces
- 1 celery stalk, cut into ½-inch pieces
- 4 cups chopped leeks, white parts only
- 1 cup vegetable stock
- 1 carrot, chopped
- 4 garlic cloves, minced
- 2 bay leaves
- Salt and black pepper to taste
- 2 cups heavy cream
- ¼ cup chopped fresh chives

Directions

Prepare a water bath and place the Sous Vide in it. Set to 186 F. Place the potatoes, carrots, onion, celery, leeks, vegetable stock, butter, garlic, and bay leaves in a vacuum-sealable bag. Release air by the water displacement method, seal, and submerge the bag in the water bath. Cook for 2 hours.

Once the timer has stopped, remove the bag and transfer into a blender. Discard the bay leaves. Mix the contents and season with salt and pepper. Pour the cream slowly and blend 2-3 minutes until smooth. Drain the contents and garnish with chives to serve.

47. Cheesy Bell Peppers with Cauliflower

Prep + Cook Time: 52 minutes | Servings: 5

Ingredients

- ½ cup shaved Provolone cheese
- 1 head cauliflower, cut florets
- 2 garlic cloves, minced
- Salt and black pepper to taste
- 2 tbsp butter
- 1 tbsp olive oil
- ½ large red bell pepper, cut strips
- ½ yellow bell pepper, cut into strips
- ½ orange bell pepper, cut into strips

Directions

Prepare a water bath and place the Sous Vide in it. Set to 186 F. Combine well the cauliflower florets, 1 clove of garlic, salt, pepper, half of butter, and half of olive oil. In another bowl, mix the bell peppers, remaining garlic, remaining salt, pepper, remaining butter, and remaining olive oil. Place the cauliflower in a vacuum-sealable bag. Place the bell peppers in another vacuum-sealable bag. Release air by the water displacement method, seal and submerge the bags in the water bath. Cook for 40 minutes.

Once the timer has stopped, remove the bags and transfer the contents into a serving bowl. Discard the cooking juices. Combine the vegetables and top with Provolone cheese.

48.   Herby Mashed Snow Peas

Prep + Cook Time: 55 minutes | Servings: 6

Ingredients

- ½ cup vegetable broth
- 1 pound fresh snow peas
- Zest of 1 lemon
- 2 tbsp chopped fresh basil
- 1 tbsp olive oil
- Salt and black pepper to taste
- 2 tbsp chopped fresh chives
- 2 tbsp chopped fresh parsley
- ¾ tsp garlic powder

Directions

Prepare a water bath and place the Sous Vide in it. Set to 186 F. Combine the peas, lemon zest, basil, olive oil, black pepper, chives, parsley, salt, and garlic powder and place them in a vacuum-sealable bag. Release air by the water displacement method, seal, and submerge the bag in the water bath. Cook for 45 minutes. Once the timer has stopped, remove the bag and transfer into a blender and mix well.

49. Buttered Asparagus with Thyme & Cheese

Prep + Cook Time: 21 minutes | Servings: 6

Ingredients

- ¼ cup shaved Pecorino Romano cheese
- 16 oz fresh asparagus, trimmed
- 4 tbsp butter, cubed
- Salt to taste
- 1 garlic clove, minced
- 1 tbsp thyme

Directions

Prepare a water bath and place the Sous Vide in it. Set to 186 F. Place the asparagus in a vacuum-sealable bag. Add the butter cubes, garlic, salt, and thyme. Release air by the water displacement method, seal, and submerge the bag in the water bath. Cook for 14 minutes. Once the timer has stopped, transfer the asparagus to a plate. Top with cooking juices. Garnish with Pecorino Romano cheese.

50. Fall Squash Cream Soup

Prep + Cook Time: 2 hours 20 minutes | Servings: 6

Ingredients

- ¾ cup heavy cream
- 1 winter squash, chopped
- 1 large pear
- ½ yellow onion, diced
- 3 fresh thyme sprigs
- 1 garlic clove, chopped
- 1 tsp ground cumin
- Salt and black pepper to taste
- 4 tbsp crème fraîche

Directions

Prepare a water bath and place the Sous Vide in it. Set to 186 F. Combine the squash, pear, onion, thyme, garlic, cumin, and salt. Place in a vacuum-sealable bag. Release air by the water displacement method, seal and submerge in the water bath. Cook for 2 hours. Once the timer has stopped, remove the bag and transfer all the contents into a blender. Puree until smooth. Add in cream and stir well. Season with salt and pepper. Transfer the mix into serving bowls and top with some créme fraiche. Garnish with pear chunks.

CHAPTER 9.   Desserts & Drinks

51.Fresh Fruit Créme Brulée

Prep + Cook Time: 65 minutes + 5 hours Cooling Time | Servings: 6

Ingredients

- 1 cup fresh blackberries
- 6 egg yolks
- 1⅓ cups sugar + more for sprinkling
- 3 cups heavy cream
- Zest of 2 orange
- 4 tbsp orange juice
- 1 tsp vanilla extract

Directions

Prepare a water bath and place the Sous Vide in it. Set to 196 F. In a blender, mix the egg yolks and sugar until creamy. Set aside. Heat a saucepan over medium heat and pour the cream. Add the orange zest and juice and vanilla extract. Lower the heat and cook for 4-5 minutes. Put the blackberries in six mason jars, pour the egg-cream mixture over the blackberries. Seal with a lid and submerge the jars in the water bath. Cook for 45 minutes.

Once the timer has stopped, remove the jars and transfer into the fridge and allow to chill for 5 hours. Remove the lid and sprinkle with sugar. Caramelize the sugar with a blowtorch.

52.   Vanilla Berry Pudding

Prep + Cook Time: 2 hours 32 minutes | Servings: 6

Ingredients

- 1 cup mixed fresh berries
- 4 slices challah, cubed
- 6 egg yolks
- 1⅛ cups superfine sugar
- 2 cups heavy cream
- 1 cup milk
- T2 sp almond extract
- 1 vanilla pod, halved, seeds reserved

Directions

Prepare a water bath and place the Sous Vide in it. Set to 172 F. Preheat the oven to 350 F. Place bread cubes in a baking tray and toast for 5 minutes. Set aside. With an electric mixer, mix the egg yolks and sugar until creamy.Heat a saucepan over medium heat and pour in cream and milk. Cook until boiled. Add in almond extract, vanilla pod seeds and vanilla pod. Lower the heat and cook for 4-5 minutes. Set aside and allow to cool for 2-3 minutes. Once the vanilla mixture has cooled, pour a small amount of the cream into the egg mixture and combine. Repeat the process with each egg. Combine the bread cubes with the egg-cream mixture and let the bread absorb the liquid. Add the berries and combine well. Divide the mixture into six mason jars. Seal with a lid and submerge the jars in the water bath. Cook for 2 hours.

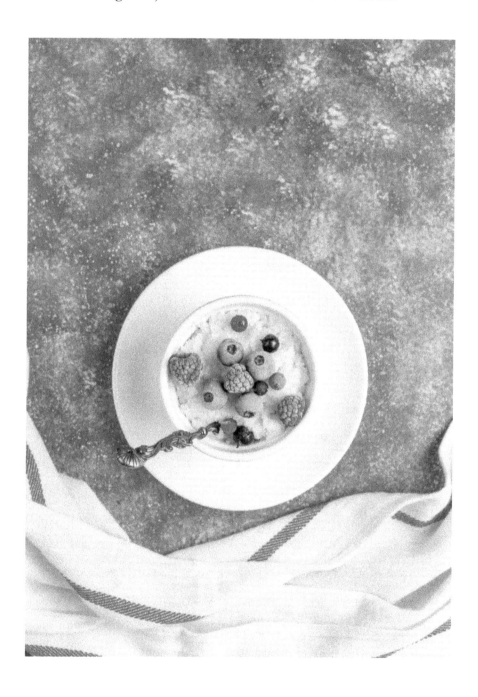

53.   Mocha Mini Brownies in a Jar

Prep + Cook Time: 3 hours 17 minutes | Servings: 10

Ingredients

- ⅔ cup white chocolate, chopped
- 8 tbsp butter
- ⅔ cup superfine sugar
- 2 egg yolks
- 1 egg
- 2 tbsp instant coffee powder
- 1 tbsp coconut extract
- 1 tbsp coffee liqueur
- ½ cup all-purpose flour
- Ice cream, for serving

Directions

Prepare a water bath and place Sous Vide in it. Set to 196 F. Heat the chocolate and butter in a pot or in the microwave. Fold sugar into the chocolate-butter mixture until dissolved. Pour the egg yolks one by one and stir well. Add in whole egg and continue mixing. Pour in coffee powder, coconut extract and coffee liqueur.

Add in flour and stir until combined well. Pour the chocolate mixture into 10 mini mason jars. Seal with a lid and submerge the jars in the water bath. Cook for 3 hours. Once ready, remove the jars and allow to cool for 1 minute.

54. Orange Pots du Créme with Chocolate

Prep + Cook Time: 6 hours 5 minutes + | Servings: 6

Ingredients

- ⅔ cup chopped chocolate
- 6 egg yolks
- 1⅓ cups fine white sugar
- 3 cups half and half
- 1 tsp vanilla extract
- Zest of 1 large orange
- ⅛ tsp orange extract
- 2 tbsp orange juice
- 2 tbsp chocolate-flavored liqueur

Directions

Prepare a water bath and place the Sous Vide in it. Set to 196 F. With an electric mixer, combine the egg yolks and sugar. Mix for 1-2 minutes until creamy. Heat the cream in a saucepan over medium heat and add in vanilla, orange zest and extract. Cook on Low heat for 3-4 minutes. Set aside and allow to cool for 2-3 minutes.

Melt the chocolate in the microwave. Once the mixture has cooled, pour the cream mixture into the egg mixture and stir. Add the melted chocolate and stir until combined. Add in orange juice and chocolate liqueur. Pour the chocolate mixture into mason jars. Seal with a lid and submerge the jars in the water bath. Cook for 45 minutes. Once the timer has stopped, remove the jars and allow to cool for 5 minutes.

55.   Vanilla Ice Cream

Prep + Cook Time: 5 hours 10 minutes | Servings: 4

Ingredients

- 6 egg yolks
- ½ cup sugar
- 1 ½ tsp vanilla extract
- 2 cups half and half

Directions

Prepare a water bath and place the Sous Vide in it. Set to 180 F. Whisk all the ingredients in a vacuum-sealable bag. Release air by the water displacement method, seal, and submerge the bag in the water bath. Set the timer for 1 hour. Once the timer has stopped, make sure there are no lumps. Transfer the mixture to a container with a lid. Place in the freeze for 4 hours.

56.   Chocolate Pudding

Prep + Cook Time: 55 minutes | Servings: 4

Ingredients

- ½ cup milk
- cup chocolate chips
- 3 egg yolks
- ½ cup heavy cream
- 4 tbsp cocoa powder
- tbsp sugar

Directions

Prepare a water bath and place the Sous Vide in it. Set to 185 F. Whisk the yolks along with sugar, milk, and heavy cream. Stir in cocoa powder and chocolate chips. Divide the mixture between 4 jars. Seal and immerse the jars in the water bath. Set the timer for 40 minutes. Once ready, remove the jars. Let cool before serving.

57.   Honey & Citrus Apricots

Prep + Cook Time: 70 minutes | Servings: 4

Ingredients

- 6 apricots, pitted and quartered
- ½ cup honey
- 2 tbsp water
- 1 tbsp lime juice
- 1 vanilla bean pod, halved
- 1 cinnamon stick

Directions

Prepare a water bath and place the Sous Vide in it. Set to 179 F. Place all the ingredients in a vacuum-sealable bag. Release air by the water displacement method, seal, and submerge the bag in the water bath. Cook for 45 minutes. Once the timer has stopped, remove the bag and discard the vanilla bean pod and cinnamon stick. Serve.

58.   Light Cottage Cheese Breakfast Pudding

Prep + Cook Time: 3 hours 15 minutes | Servings: 3

Ingredients

- 1 cup cottage cheese
- 5 eggs
- cup milk - 3 tbsp sour cream
- 4 tbsp sugar
- tsp cardamom
- 1 tsp orange zest 1 tbsp cornstarch ¼ tsp salt

Directions

Prepare a water bath and place Sous Vide in it. Set to 175 F. With an electric mixer, beat the eggs and sugar. Add in zest, milk and cornstarch. Add the remaining ingredients and whisk well.

Grease 3 mason jars with cooking spray and divide the mixture between them. Seal and immerse the mason jars in a water bath. Cook for 3 hours. Once the timer has stopped, remove the jars. Let cool before serving.

59.   Sous Vide Chocolate Cupcakes

Prep + Cook Time: 3 hours 15 minutes | Servings: 6

Ingredients

- 5 tbsp butter, melted
- 1 egg
- 3 tbsp cocoa powder
- 1 cup flour
- 4 tbsp sugar
- ½ cup heavy cream
- 1 tsp baking soda
- 1 tsp vanilla extract
- 1 tsp apple cider vinegar
- Pinch of sea salt

Directions

Prepare a water bath and place the Sous Vide in it. Set to 194 F. Whisk together the wet ingredients in one bowl. Combine the dry ingredients in another bowl. Combine the two mixtures gently and divide the batter between 6 small jars. Seal the jars and submerge the bag in the water bath. Set the timer for 3 hours Once the timer has stopped, remove the bag. Serve chilled.

60.   Sous Vide Limoncello

Prep + Cook Time: 3 hours 8 minutes | Servings: 6

Ingredients

- 14 ounces vodka
- Zest of 3 lemons 2 ounces sugar

Directions

Prepare a water bath and place the Sous Vide in it. Set to 130 F. Place all the ingredients in a mason jar. Seal and submerge in the water bath. Set the timer for 3 hours. Once the timer has stopped, remove the bag. Serve with ice.